VEGAN

30 Days of Vegan Recipes and Meal Plans for Increasing Your Health and Energy

© **Copyright 2016 - All rights reserved.**

The contents of this book may not be reproduced, duplicated or transmitted without direct written permission from the author.

Under no circumstances will any legal responsibility or blame be held against the publisher for any reparation, damages, or monetary loss due to the information herein, either directly or indirectly.

Legal Notice:
This book is copyright protected. This is only for personal use. You cannot amend, distribute, sell, use, quote or paraphrase any part or the content within this book without the consent of the author.

Disclaimer Notice:
Please note the information contained within this document is for educational and entertainment purposes only. Every attempt has been made to provide accurate, up to date and reliable complete information. No warranties of any kind are expressed or implied. Readers acknowledge that the author is not engaging in the rendering of legal, financial, medical or professional advice. The content of this book has been derived from various sources. Please consult a licensed professional before attempting any techniques outlined in this book.

By reading this document, the reader agrees that under no circumstances are is the author responsible for any losses, direct or indirect, which are incurred as a result of the use of information contained within this document, including, but not limited to, —errors, omissions, or inaccuracies.

Free membership into the Mastermind Self Development Group!

For a limited time, you can join the Mastermind Self Development Group for free! You will receive videos and articles from top authorities in self development as well as a special group only offers on new books and training programs. There will also be a monthly member only draw that gives you a chance to win any book from your Kindle wish list!

If you sign up through this link http://www.mastermindselfdevelopment.com/specialreport you will also get a special free report on the Wheel of Life. This report will give you a visual look at your current life and then take you through a series of exercises that will help you plan what your perfect life looks like. The workbook does not end there; we then take you through a process to help you plan how to achieve that perfect life. The process is very powerful and has the potential to change your life forever. Join the group now and start to change your life!
http://www.mastermindselfdevelopment.com/specialreport

Table of Contents

Introduction

Chapter 1: Why to Go Vegan

Chapter 2: Understanding Vegan Diets

Chapter 3: Meal Plan and Outline Recipes for Block I
- **Day 1**
- **Day 2**
- **Day 3**
- **Day 4**
- **Day 5**
- **Day 6**
- **Day 7**
- **Day 8**

Chapter 4: Meal Plan and Outline Recipes for Block II
- **Day 9**
- **Day 10**
- **Day 11**
- **Day 12**
- **Day 13**
- **Day 14**
- **Day 15**
- **Day 16**

Chapter 5: Meal Plan and Recipes for Block III
- **Day 17**
- **Day 18**
- **Day 19**
- **Day 20**
- **Day 21**
- **Day 22**
- **Day 23**

Chapter 6: Meal Plan and Recipes for Block IV
- **Day 24**
- **Day 25**
- **Day 26**
- **Day 27**
- **Day 28**
- **Day 29**
- **Day 30**

Conclusion – How to Stay Committed

Introduction

Veganism is fast catching up with many people across the world. The noble idea behind veganism such as not wanting to exploit the less fortunate animal species of the world by taking what is theirs and selfishly using it for ourselves simply because they do not have the power to stop us is, perhaps, the primary reason for the growth in popularity of this concept.

However, in addition to the above extremely thoughtful reason, the health benefits and other great things about veganism are all sufficiently powerful causes for the expansion of the idea of veganism across the planet. This book is written with an intention to exhort newcomers to try a one-month vegan challenge that has the power to change not just your lifestyle but your entire outlook on life.

Before you decide to try to change your lifestyle to vegan, there are a few things you must know and understand about it. This book aims to do exactly that by giving you a detailed overview in the following areas:

- What is veganism?
- A brief history on veganism
- How is veganism useful to you?
- Meal Plans for a one-month challenge along with recipe outlines
- How to stay committed to the cause?

What is veganism?

You know who are vegetarians? They do not consume poultry, meat, or, fish in their diet. Vegans, additionally, do not consume or use any animal products and/or by-products such as dairy products, honey, eggs, leather, silk, fur, and soaps and cosmetics made from animal sources. Vegans are the superset of vegetarians. All vegans are also vegetarians but all vegetarians need not be vegans.

Vegans believe that veganism is not just about their diet but a way of life. As far as possible, vegans avoid exploitation of animals in any form including but not limited to food, clothing, or other purposes. They also avoid items that have been tested on animals before being commercialized. And believe it or not, there is a vegan diet for all kinds of diets ranging from the junk food lovers to the raw food lovers and those in between, too.

History of Veganism

Veganism, although not known as veganism, has been around for many centuries. Examples of prevention of exploitation against and cruelty to animals have been written in history books. Lord Buddha of India and Pythagoras both advocated this concept and had put in rules to ensure their followers ate only plant-based food and completely avoided meats and animal products.

The earliest modern-day veganism is known to have occurred around 1806 CE. During that time, the great English poet P B Shelley and Dr. William Lambe publicly objected to consuming dairy products and eggs by humans on ethical grounds. This incident seems to have laid the foundation for modern-day veganism.

In November 1944, six non-dairy vegetarians including Donald Watson and Elsie Shrigley called met together and discussed the topic on non-dairy vegetarians' lifestyles and diets. Despite strong opposition, these six members founded the new movement and became actively involved in this new project.

When the Vegan Society was formalized and registered as a charity organization in 1979, the Memorandum and Articles of Association of the society defined veganism as:

"...a philosophy and way of living which seeks to exclude – as far as possible and practicable – all forms of exploitation of, and cruelty to, animals for food, clothing or any other purpose; and by extension, promotes the development and use of animal-free alternatives for the benefit of humans, animals, and the environment. In dietary terms, it denotes the practice of dispensing with all products derived wholly or partly from animals."

This book deals only with the dietary aspect of veganism giving you amply sufficient reasons to shift your lifestyle to this healthy and noble one. While the benefits of turning vegan are discussed in another chapter, the kind of foods that you can include in your diet while keeping your energy levels and health not just unchanged but also improved than earlier is huge.

Here is a small list of foods that are known to be totally vegan:

- All kinds of grains and cereals
- All kinds of beans and legumes

- All fruits and vegetables

Other vegan foods include soy milk, vegan mayonnaise, vegan ice cream and cheese, vegan hot dogs, and more. Moreover, a lot of companies have come out with mock meats that give vegans a sense of eating meat. This book also has 4 chapters dedicated to making vegan foods, which includes easy-to-make recipes.

Chapter 1: Why to Go Vegan

Most people in the world want to do the following things by some means or the other:

- Lose weight
- Eat better
- Get fitter and healthier
- Do something for society and the world at large

The great news is that if you shift to a vegan diet, you can achieve all the above goals. And let me assure you, you will enjoy delicious, wholesome, and satiating meals as well.

No loss or reduction in energy levels – There is a misconception that changing to vegan diet reduces your energy levels. There are numerous unworthy talks of vegans living only on water and a few greens and hence their energy levels have taken a huge dip. And on the other side of the spectrum, there are plenty of spurious rumors that talk of people going vegan is helping them do impossible things. These other-end-of-the-spectrum talks make out vegans to be people who can walk on water! Let me assure you that neither of the extremes is true or based on any scientific studies.

Health benefits are huge when you choose to go vegan. Of course, the initial learning curve is going to be steep and you would have to counter multiple challenges. However, once you have overcome these tough phases and complete the 30-day challenge, you are going feel to fitter, lighter, and happier. Moreover, there are multiple studies done by various organizations including the British Dietetic Association that has proven the excellent efficacies of getting fitter and healthier by following a vegan diet.

Here is the list of a few magic foods that can restore energy instantaneously:

Bananas – Already beautifully and naturally packaged by nature, this wonderful tropical fruit is normally the first you must reach out for when you feel tired or fatigued.

Walnuts – Another great pick-me-up tree nut, walnuts are rich in plant proteins, omega fatty acids, and vitamins giving you the almost-instant energy boost.

Green smoothies – Delicious smoothies made by tossing together strawberries, bananas, and orange juices are great and extremely healthy pick-me-ups to fight fatigue.

Coconut water – This is nature's energy drink and is amazingly refreshing and is filled with vitamins and potassium.

Kiwi – This low-fat delicious fruit is an instant energy enhancer triggered by the simple sugars present in it.

Why I chose to mention vegan energy boosters in the beginning itself is to help you overcome doubts regarding your ability to get on with your daily schedule if you choose to go vegan. Today there are many sportspeople who have shifted to this diet to keep fitter and sustain energy levels. So, if highly active people in the field of sports can take advantage of veganism, it should not be difficult for moderately active people like us to take this 30-day challenge and come out with flying colors.

Other great reasons to take the one-month challenge to go vegan are:

Lose weight and yet remain energized – Many of us love to find a sensible way to lose excess weight and yet remain healthy and fit. Average vegans are known to weigh 20 pounds lesser than average meat-eaters. Despite this, vegan diets do not starve you and make you feel enervated like the usual run-of-the-meal fad diets do.

Keep diseases and health disorders away – The Academy of Nutrition and Dietetics have conducted multiple studies which show that taking the vegan route helps you steer clear of common disorders such as diabetes, hypertension or high blood pressure thereby preventing the onset of many modern-day diseases such as heart attacks, kidney failure, and others.

Vegan foods are yummy and delicious – If you thought going vegan means you would have to give up your favorite ice creams, hamburgers, and chicken sandwiches, then you are wrong. With demand for vegan products soaring, many companies are coming up with amazingly delicious vegan options that taste very much like the non-vegetarian stuff. You will not miss any of the meats and animal products at all. There are plenty of established brands that cater to veganism and deliver really tasty dairy and meat substitutes.

Vegan diets are full of highly nutritious and healthy food items including whole grains, beans and legumes, nuts, soy products, and fresh fruits and vegetables. Here are some of the health benefits that these fiber-rich and healthy food sources provide you with:

- **Minimal saturated fats** – Meats and dairy products contain plenty of saturated fats thereby increasing the risk of cardiovascular diseases. Vegan diets automatically reduce intake of saturated fats enhancing your health condition

- **Fiber** – A vegan diet is high in fiber content that is very conducive to healthy bowel movements.

- **Magnesium** – Dark, green leafy vegetables are a rich source of magnesium, a key element that aids the body in the absorption of calcium.

- **Potassium** – Similarly, potassium, an important mineral that balances acidity and water in our body and helps in the removal of toxins is found in plenty in plant-based foods.

- **Proteins** – Meat-eaters invariably end up with more proteins than is needed by the body. Vegan diets, which include nuts, beans, and legumes, have the right amount of proteins for us.

Vegan diets provide other critically essential nutrients such as Vitamins E and C, phytochemicals, antioxidants, and foliates. These help in keeping your immunity system healthy and robust and also prevent age-related diseases such as Alzheimer's and Parkinson's disease and keep your overall body organs functioning well.

Vegan diets have the power to prevent the following diseases that are very common in today's high-stressed unhealthy lifestyle:

- Cardiovascular diseases
- Reduced cholesterol due to the complete absence of meat and dairy products in your diet
- Age-related macular degeneration
- Reduced risk of breast cancer

- Reduced risk of contracting ailments like diabetes, hypertension, cataracts, colon and prostate cancer, arthritis, and osteoporosis

In addition to improved health and prevention of diseases, going vegan makes you stronger, more energetic, and more attractive. Here is how:

Lowered Body Mass Index – A diet without meat and dairy products automatically help in the reduction of body mass index

Weight loss – Weight loss is an unquestioned effect of a vegan diet.

Healthy skin – Consuming rich sources of Vitamins A and E from nuts and fruits and vegetables enhance the texture and health of your skin.

Reduced allergy symptoms – Plant-based foods do not trigger as many allergic reactions in humans as dairy and meat products do.

Less intake of mercury – A lot of shellfish and fish contain high levels of mercury, which we take in when we eat these foods. Switching to veganism does away with this toxin completely.

The above are only some of the great reasons that you must start off this 30-day vegan challenge. Instead of finding reasons not to do something good, focus on the above reasons which tell you why you should do it and dive straight in. Summon some extra willpower from yourself and after you complete this challenge you can rest assured that the willpower would come on its own when you see and feel the wondrous new VEGAN YOU.

Chapter 2: Understanding Vegan Diets

In the previous chapter, along with why should you go vegan, I had mentioned some basic foods that can deliver instant energy whenever you feel enervated. Just to reiterate, the foods listed are all completely vegan and yet are employed by all to get back energy levels when they feel sapped.

Considering the huge amount of misconception, doubts, and skepticism regarding energy levels and maintenance of good health by vegan, I thought it made sense to dedicate one chapter to help you overcome these misunderstandings which in turn will, I hope, will catapult your move to try out the 30-day vegan challenge.

There are many ex-vegans who complain of fogginess, depression, and other challenging mental and social circumstances when they chose to give up animal foods. Understanding the power and function of each nutrient is highly helpful in managing those seemingly difficult days especially during the initial days when support system and a common social network help you understand the root cause the issues and get you an objective and tried-and-tested solution.

Knowing how the various nutrients derived from animal and plant sources differ from each other, which vegan foods give you optimum results and how to keep feelings of depression due to short-term failures at bay are all critical elements in making a success of your 30-day vegan challenge. And when you come out successful in a small attempt, you will be emboldened to try for something bigger.

Carbohydrates for vegans – Cutting back on carbohydrates for anyone is not that difficult for anyone including for us vegans. It is essential for you to use low-carb food sources to maintain good health with a vegan diet.

Vegetables: There are many vegetables which are low-carb foods including onions, tomatoes, eggplant, cauliflower, broccoli, bell peppers, and more.

Fruits: Blueberries and strawberries are low-carb foods. However, depending on how much you need daily, other fruits can easily be included.

Fatty foods – Olives and avocados are high in good fats and low-carb too and hence excellent dietary inclusions for vegans.

Soy, nuts, and seeds: These are low in carbohydrates and high in fats and proteins. So, it is imperative to include soy, soy-based foods, nuts, and seeds into your daily diet.

Chia seeds: I deliberately included this one special item because most of the carbohydrates in chia seeds are in the form of fiber. Hence, most of the energy source from this food is got from fats and proteins. Do include chia seeds whenever you can.

Additionally, choose slow carbohydrate foods, that is, consume carb sources that have a low glycemic index. These foods prevent high fluctuations in your blood sugar levels and you will feel more satiated over a longer period as they release glucose slowly. For instance, choose breads that have been made from non-ground grains, use barley, quinoa, and oats in place of rice, use fresh beans and legumes instead of canned ones, use sweet potatoes instead of white potatoes.

Animal Protein Vs. Plant Protein – As our body does not accumulate protein, it is imperative that we take in proteins in our daily diet. Proteins are available both in plant-based and animal-based foods. The different between the two sources is the profile of amino acid present. Amino acids are of different types (about 20 of them are very critical for us) and all of them are essential for carrying out multiple metabolic activities in our body.

Animal proteins invariably have a sufficiently wide of range of amino acids in them whereas many plant proteins are not complete. For instance, many plant proteins are quite low in important amino acids such as tryptophan, methionine, isoleucine, and lysine, Legumes, on the other hand, are the best plant-based protein source that is comparable to meats. For this express reason, ensure you eat 3 servings of legumes daily in the form of peas, beans, peanuts, tofu etc. This will keep you energy levels optimum and considerably reduce your craving for meats.

Fats in vegan diets – Very low-fat foods are not great for vegan diets. In fact, a lot of recent studies have proved that very low-fat diets are not effective in the long-term. However, a free-for-all fatty diet is also an absolute no-no. It is important to include good-fat foods such as nuts and avocados to get the right quality and quantity of fat. Nutrition experts believe you should consume not more than 30 gm. of saturated fats every day.

Vitamins, Omega-3 fats, and other important nutrients – Animal protein foods contain higher levels and a wider range of other important nutrients such as Vitamins (B12 and D), DHA (Docosahexaenoic acid), which is an essential omega-3 fatty acid, zinc, and heme-iron. The four listed nutrients are found in abundance in meats such as pork, beef, dairy products, eggs, and fish, but are a little low in plant-based foods.

While this may seem a concern, let me assure you that there are ample solutions for this other than simply giving up a fantastically healthy lifestyle that has the power to change multiple things in a positive way (already discussed in the previous chapter). Omega-3 fatty acids are available in plenty in walnuts, flaxseed and flaxseed oil, and chia seeds. Vitamin B12 plant-based analogs include sourdough bread, fermented soy foods, shiitake mushrooms, and sea vegetables. Moreover, these trace nutritional elements like Vitamin B12, Vitamin D, iodine etc. can be easily taken as supplements.

Most plant-based foods are rich in folate (dark, green leafy veggies provide this nutrient in plenty), potassium, calcium (figs, nuts, almonds etc. are wonderfully rich in calcium), iron (lentils are a great source) Vitamin C, phytochemicals, and Vitamin A (carrots). So these nutrients are well covered in a vegan diet through the intake of ample amounts of differently colored fruits and vegetables.

Do not hesitate to use convenience foods – There are plenty of convenience products for vegans available in the market today. These include vegan ice creams, vegan meats, and vegan cheeses. When you are pressed for time and need convenience over laborious cooking processes, do not hesitate to use these options as they will go a long way in helping you stay committed to the vegan cause especially in the early days when you are still in the learning curve.

Chapter 3: Meal Plan and Outline Recipes for Block I

The next few chapters are dedicated to giving you meal plans along with some basic recipes for the start of your 30-day vegan challenge journey.

Day 1

Green smoothies for Breakfast – In a blender, mix mango juice and coconut water till the two are smoothly blended. Now add parsley, cilantro, avocado, and ice cubes and blend again to get a thick super smooth smoothie. Adjust tartness and sweetness levels to match your liking.

Lemon and Citrus Couscous with Fennel and Chickpeas for Lunch – In a pan, cook the trimmed fennel for till caramelized. To this, add cooked chickpeas, ground coriander, lemon juice, and olives and continue cooking for a medium flame till you a nice veggie-filled sauce. To give the couscous a citrusy flavor, cook it in a mixture of orange juice and water along with some lemon and orange zest, a little olive oil, and salt. To serve this couscous meal, fluff up the couscous using a fork. Make a layer of the couscous plate and over it, spoon out the fennel and chickpeas mixture. You can now use the fennel frond for garnishing. Dig into your delicious vegan lunch.

Tofu-Spinach Lasagna for Dinner - Cook the lasagna noodles as directed on the package, drain and keep aside. Squeeze the spinach to remove water as much as possible. In a blender, blitz together sugar, tofu, soymilk, lemon juice, garlic powder, salt, and basil till you get a smooth blend. Now, stir in the dried spinach. Take a baking dish and make a layer of tomato sauce at the bottom. Make a layer of the cooked lasagna noodles over this and over this a layer of the tofu mixture. Repeat the three layers again till all the materials are used up. The top layer should be that of the noodles and tomato sauce poured over it. In a preheated oven, bake this for about 25-30 minutes.

Day 2

Mango Smoothie for Breakfast - Add 2 cups frozen mango, 1 ½ cup orange juice, ½ cup avocado, ½ tsp lime zest, pure maple syrup (to taste), and appropriate amount of water into a blender and blitz together everything till you get a lovely, thick, and creamy smoothie

Avocado and sauerkraut sandwiches for lunch - Spread Dijon mustard on one slice of pumpernickel or rye bread and spread Thousand Island vegan dressing on the other slice. On an oiled (lightly) skillet, place the two slices (dry side down) and grill till golden brown. Pile on sauerkraut topping for one slice and avocado on the other slice. Continue to grill over medium heat for about 5 minutes. Remove from heat and join two halves and enjoy. Combine with cucumber and tomato salad for a complete vegan meal

Scallion Pancakes for Dinner - Make pancake dough with all-purpose flour, knead well and keep aside for some time. Then roll out the dough (1/8-inch thickness); spread a layer of vegetable shortening, and then sprinkle a layer of salt and then a layer of green onions. Gently roll this into a jelly-shaped roll and cut out fist-sized pieces. Again, with rolling pin, roll out each piece into 1/8-inch thick slices and cook on an oiled skillet till both sides for about 2 minutes each. Place the cooked pancakes on paper tissues to remove the excess oil and dig in. You could use soy sauce as a tartar dip.

Day 3

Chocolate Hemp Smoothie for Breakfast – In a blender add almond milk (2 cups), 2-3 pitted dates, 3 tbsp. unsweetened cocoa powder, 3 tbsp. hemp seeds (hulled), 1 banana (peeled and cut into slices/cubes), ¼ tsp cinnamon powder, and ice cubes. Blend it all together till the mixture reaches a thick, creamy, and smoothie-like (though this will be of a slightly thinner consistency) consistency. Pour into a glass and drink away

Minestrone Soup and Crusty Bread for Lunch – In a saucepan, heat 1 tbsp. of olive oil (extra virgin) over medium heat. Sauté ¾ cup finely chopped onions, and add the following water, diced zucchini, carrots, beans, canned tomatoes, minced garlic, diced celery, dried basil, and pepper, oregano, and salt. Bring all this to a boil, and simmer for about 25-30 minutes till all ingredients are cooked. Now add ¼ cup macaroni and cook for another 10 minutes. Adjust spices to your taste and serve hot with some pumpernickel or rye bread (roasted on a skillet with a dash of oil).

Vegan sausages for dinner - Get your steaming apparatus ready with water brought to a full boil. Cool and mash beans nicely till no lumps are left. Add olive oil, soy sauce, finely minced garlic, wheat gluten, nutritional yeast, crushed fennel seeds, red pepper flakes, pepper, oregano, and salt and mix well till you get nice smooth dough-like consistency. Divide this dough into 4-6 portions and make each portion into a log shape (like the meat sausages). Place these on separate tin foils and roll the foil to look like a tootsie roll. Put these wrapped vegan sausages in the steamer and cook for about 40 minutes. Remove from heat and your vegan sausages are ready. Serve hot with a nice soy sauce dip or simply with ketchup.

Day 4

Peanut Butter Banana Smoothie for Breakfast – In a blender, add 2 sliced frozen bananas, 4 small dates, 1 tbsp. peanut butter, 1 tbsp. chia seeds, and ¼ cup water. Blitz together and your smoothie is ready.

Asparagus, Potato, and Squash Frittata for Lunch - Fry the squash and potatoes till golden brown. To this add garlic, dried herbs, and onions and continue to sauté till the onions are soft. Add salt and pepper for seasoning. Now, put in the asparagus and stir for a couple more minutes. Put this veggie mixture into cake tin. In a blender, blitz together tofu and other remaining ingredients (except the dried herbs) until smooth. Now add the herbs and mix well. Pour this tofu mixture onto the veggie layer. Smoothen out the tofu layer with a knife and bake for 30-40 minutes in a medium heat oven.

Tempeh Casserole for Dinner - Mash the tempeh either in a food processor or with a potato masher. In a big bowl, mix this mashed tempeh with onions, zucchini, broccoli stock, brown rice, arrowroot starch, balsamic vinegar, herbs, baking powder, and egg substitute and place in a casserole. In a preheated oven at 350F, cook for about 20 minutes. For the sauce, combine vegan mayo, paprika, and salt.

Day 5

Strawberry and Avocado Smoothie for Breakfast – In a food processor, blend together ½ a frozen banana, 2 cups of fresh strawberries, 3 tbsp. of spearmint, 1 ½ cups of coconut water, ½ an avocado, 1 pitted date, and ice cubes. Your smoothie is ready to drink.

Adzuki Bean Burgers with Potato Wedges for Lunch - Boil the water in a saucepan and add a packet of oats. Simmer for about 2 minutes till the oats are cooked. Over a medium flame, heat 2 tbsp. of olive oil and put in celery, onions, garlic, and carrots and cook until tender. Add a little water, salt and basil to this mixture and stir occasionally and cook for another 5 minutes.

In a food processor, blitz together the onion mixture, cooked oats, adzuki beans, and parsley. Stir in the brown rice flour till you get a dough-like consistency that can be molded into patties. Form 8-10 patties with this. Cook the patties on a skillet with a dash of oil. Place between toasted pumpernickel or rye bread and enjoy your meal.

Lentil and Barley Casserole for Dinner - In a large pan, heat oil and sauté the onions and garlic. Add potatoes, swede, and carrots (all cut into large chunks) and continue cooking till the veggies get tender. Put in rosemary, bay leaves, thyme, and tomato paste. Pour 5 cups of water and add pearl barley, lentils, stock powder, stock cube, and mushrooms. Add a little pepper for seasoning. Bring this mixture to a boil and then simmer over a low flame for about 45 minutes till a casserole constituency is achieved. Remove the bay leaves and then serve.

Day 6

Cherry limeade Smoothie for Breakfast – In a blender, blend together 1 ripe peach (sliced), 1 cup frozen cherries, ¾ cup almond milk, juice of 1 lime, and some ice cubes. Your smoothie is ready.

Baked Potatoes and Coleslaw for Lunch - Smear a little olive oil on the washed and dried potatoes and bake in a preheated oven for about 1 to 1 ½ hours till soft on the inside and crisp on the outside. For the coleslaw, combine cream cheese, vegan mayonnaise, and mustard till you get a smooth mixture. Add this to finely chopped cabbage, carrots, and onions, and mix well. Season as needed and refrigerate. When the potatoes are ready, cut in the middle and add the coleslaw and serve.

Noodles with vegetables and tofu for dinner - In a small bowl, mix together soy sauce, sweet chili sauce, and vegetarian mushroom sauce. In a large bowl, put a packet of noodles and cover completely with hot water. Close with a lid and set aside. Heat olive oil in a saucepan or wok and stir fry chopped onions for a minute. Now add ginger, garlic and vegetables of your choice including carrots, zucchini, red capsicum, and broccoli. Add some tofu too and fry for a further 2-3 minutes. Use 5-spice powder for seasoning. Drain the noodles. Remove all water and put it into the wok. Add the sauce mixture and mix everything well. Cook for another minute or two and serve hot.

Day 7

Creamy Chocolate Shake for Breakfast – In a blender, blitz together 2 ripe frozen bananas, 1/3 cup frozen strawberries, 2-3 tbsp. cocoa powder, 2 tbsp. almond butter (salted), 1 tbsp. flaxseed meal, 1 ½ - 2 cups almond milk or soy milk or coconut milk, a dash of agave nectar or stevia, and some ice cubes. Your shake is ready

Vegetable and Pesto Sandwich for Lunch – Roast zucchini, eggplant, capsicum, and onions along with seasoning of pepper, salt and olive oil in an oven till they turn soft and lightly brown. Spread dairy-free pesto on two bread slices and pile on the roasted veggies, tomato slices, and some lettuce leaves. Bring the slices together and your yummy sandwich is ready.

Shepherd's pie for Dinner – Boil, peel and mash some potatoes with a little salt and some vegan margarine. Sauté onions with some olive oil in a saucepan till tender and to this add chopped zucchini, mushrooms, and carrots. After the veggies have softened add tomato paste, canned tomatoes, stock cube, herbs and casserole mince and stir well. Make thick gravy with gravy powder and some water and pour into this veggie mix. Cool for about 25-30 minutes. In a baking tray, pour this veggie mixture and layer the mashed potato mix on top. Bake this dish for above 25-30 minutes till the top is nicely browned.

Day 8

5-ingredient healthy delicious smoothie for breakfast – In a blender, blitz together frozen berries, spinach, flaxseed, mixed fruit juice, and a frozen banana and your delicious breakfast smoothie is ready.

Peking Mock "duck" pancakes for lunch – Thaw the mock duck and put into a baking dish. Slather it with Peking duck sauce and bake for about 30 minutes at 200C. Shred the baked mock duck. Use readymade vegan pancake batter and cook the pancakes as directed. To serve, take a pancake, layer with Peking duck sauce, add shredded onions, cucumbers, and the mock and roll it gently. Your pancake is ready

Eggplant and Tomato Pasta for Dinner – In a large pan, add olive oil and sauté onions and minced garlic cloves. Add chopped eggplant and balsamic vinegar and cook till the veggies are soft and tender. Now add canned tomatoes, tomato paste, dried herbs, sun-dried tomatoes, chili flakes (if you like, add spice), sugar and some water. Bring this mixture to boil and cook it down for about half an hour. Cook the pasta separately and drain the excess water. Add this to the cooked veggie mixture and mix well. Add basil for improved flavor.

Chapter 4: Meal Plan and Outline Recipes for Block II

Day 9

Blueberry maple and protein shake for breakfast – In a blender, mix low-fat yogurt, 1 scoop of vanilla protein powder, ½ cup blueberries (frozen), maple extract (to taste), flaxseed meal, and some ice cubes. Your delicious and nutritious breakfast shake is ready

Veggie fritters for lunch – Mix all-purpose flour and soy milk to form batter for the fritters. Stir in sliced vegetables of your choice (zucchini, carrots, potatoes, broccoli florets, onions) and season with salt and pepper. Heat a little oil in a large skillet and spoon out a little of this mixture at a time giving it a round flat shape. Flip over and cook the other side after one side is cooked. Remove from heat, drain excess oil on tissue paper and serve hot.

Saucy tofu skewers for dinner – Cut out tofu and all your favorite veggies in roughly the same size squares. Cover with any of your favorite vegan sauces and leave to marinate for some time Barbecue or grill on a skillet till cooked. Serve with extra sauce.

Day 10

Kale-based smoothie for breakfast – In a food blender, blitz together 1 banana (medium ripe), ½ mixed berries (frozen), 1 tbsp. hulled hemp seeds, 2 cups kale leaves (fresh or frozen), 2/3 cup pomegranate juice, and some water (depending on the consistency you like; less water if you want a thick smoothie and more water if you want a thin smoothie).

Parsnip and Tempeh Rolls for lunch – Fry garlic and onions in a little oil until soft and add spices including cumin powder, dried sage, marjoram, thyme, salt and pepper and cook till the aromas are released. Add grated parsnip and tempeh to this mixture until soft. Add anchovy-free Worcestershire sauce, water, and soy sauce and cook (stirring continuously) for 4-5 minutes more till the parsnips are fully cooked. Season with salt and pepper and keep aside.

Cut pastry sheets such that you can make rectangle rolls. Place the tempeh and parsnip filling appropriately and fold over the sheet and press the meeting ends together to seal well. Then cut these filled portions into bite-sized pieces. Bake them in a preheated oven at 180C for about 15 minutes or till they are golden brown.

Chili non-carne for dinner - In a big saucepan, fry onions and garlic till soft. Add zucchini, carrots, mushrooms, and capsicum and fry some more till veggies are all tender. Add a spice mixture consisting of cumin powder, coriander powder, fennel seeds, chili flakes, peppercorns, paprika, and salt. Cook for some more time till the spices release aroma. To this add canned tomatoes, tomato paste, kidney beans (canned) and stock cube. Simmer for about half an hour and your non-carne is ready. Serve with rice, baked potatoes, enchiladas, or tacos.

Day 11

Mango Green Smoothie – In a blender, blitz together 1 ½ cups of frozen mango, 1 cup frozen strawberries, 1 cup spinach (fresh), 1 cup almond milk, and a vegan sweetener like stevia or agave. Your mango green smoothie is ready.

Spicy Couscous for lunch – In a large pan, heat some olive oil and sauté onions and garlic until translucent. Add capsicum and zucchini and cook till soft. Add spice mixture consisting of cumin, coriander, black pepper, fennel, chili flakes, and salt. Fry for another minute till the aromas of the spices are released. Stir in the couscous and add boiling water and some stock powder into this veggie mixture. Now add some sun-dried tomatoes and cooked chickpeas to this and mix thoroughly. Cover the pan with a lid and put off the heat and let it be for about 5 minutes. Once the couscous has absorbed all the stock, sprinkle some freshly chopped coriander and your lunch is ready.

Thai Red Curry for Dinner – Fry onions in a little bit of oil until tender. To this add 2 tbsp. red curry paste (ensure that the paste has no shrimp paste in it). Stir for a while and then slowly add coconut milk in small amounts stirring continuously. Now add vegetable stock. Bring this mixture to a boil and then reduce the heat to allow it to simmer.

Add tofu, mushroom, sugar, soy sauce, and capsicum to this mixture and continue to simmer for 10 more minutes. Now add bamboo shoots, chili, and sugar snap peas and cook for another 5 minutes. Serve with steamed rice.

Day 12

Mango-Strawberry with lime smoothie for breakfast – In a blender, blitz together 2 mangoes (cubed), ½ a cup frozen strawberries, lime juice (from half a lime), and ice cubes. Your lemony mango-strawberry smoothie is ready.

Asparagus and Pine Nut Tart for lunch – Cut a sheet of pastry into two such as you have 2 equal rectangles. At ½ cm from the edge, gently score the 4 sides of the pastry. Spread some mustard on the pastry sheet and place 5 asparagus sticks on each of the two rectangles (within the scored line). Bake till the pastry starts to rise. Mix together vegan cream cheese and 1 tbsp. non-dairy milk. Pour over the pastry and sprinkle some vegan cheese over. Put the pastry in the oven again and bake for about 10 minutes until golden brown. Remove from the oven and sprinkle roasted pine nuts over the tarts

Tacos and Guacamole for dinner – First make the chili non-carne (described in Day 9 dinner meal). First, heat the tacos on a skillet and then fill them with salad leaves, guacamole, salsa, and chili non-carne. Your tacos-with-guacamole meal is ready.

Day 13

Jelly Dates and Peanut butter smoothie for breakfast – In a blender, blitz together 4 medjoul dates, 1 tbsp. peanut butter, 1 frozen banana, ¾ cup almond milk, 1/3 cup frozen blueberries, and 1 tbsp. flaxseed meal. Your jelly dates and peanut butter smoothie is ready.

Pumpkin soup for lunch – In a large pan, heat oil and sauté onions and squash chunks till they start to brown. Pour boiling water till the veggies are completely covered and stir in 1 packet of noodle soup. Simmer till the squash is cooked through. Blend this entire mixture and season with salt and pepper. Serve with some crusty bread.

Marinated Tempeh Steak with Veggies for dinner – Slice the tempeh block into two thinner pieces and cut these further so that you get 4 blocks of tempeh. Marinate these tempeh blocks with garlic-infused soy sauce for as long as you can. Drizzle some oil in a skillet and fry the marinated tempeh till both the sides are brown.

For the veggies, roast pine nuts and steam the asparagus spears. Steam baby potatoes till they are soft. Toss the boiled potatoes with some vegan margarine in a hot skillet and chopped parsley. Plate the tempeh and arrange all the veggies on the side.

Day 14

Berry, Banana, and Sesame Smoothie for breakfast – Put 1 small banana, 1 tbsp. wheat germ, 4 tbsp. of sesame seeds, 5 strawberries, and 2 tbsp. of berry-flavored yogurt and blend until smooth. Pour into a glass and have a wholesome vegan breakfast

Tempeh strips with salad wraps for lunch – Marinate tempeh with garlic-infused mixtures of canola and sesame oils. After marination cut into strips and cook in a hot skillet till both sides are brown. Spread vegan margarine and beetroot dip on the ready-to-eat wraps and fill the wraps with tempeh strips and your veggies (cut into strips).

Lentil Dahl for dinner – In a saucepan, fry garlic and onions in a little bit of vegetable oil till onions are translucent. Add cumin, ginger, turmeric powder, and garam masala powder and continue to fry till the aromas of the spices are released. Now add some water, lentils, cardamom pods, stock powder, cinnamon powder, and bay leaves. Cook, while stirring occasionally, for about 25 minutes till the fully cooked. Serve hot with rice or your favorite crusty bread.

You are halfway done!

Congratulations on making it to the halfway point of the journey. Many try and give up long before even getting to this point, so you are to be congratulated on this. You have shown that you are serious about getting better every day. I am also serious about improving my life, and helping others get better along the way. To do this I need your feedback. Click on the link below and take a moment to let me know how this book has helped you. If you feel there is something missing or something you would like to see differently, I would love to know about it. I want to ensure that as you and I improve, this book continues to improve as well. Thank you for taking the time to ensure that we are all getting the most from each other.

http://viewbook.at/veganbook

Day 15

Cheesecake strawberry smoothie for breakfast – First roast the strawberries with any vegetable oil and bake for about 20 minutes till the juices of the berries are released. Now, in a blender, blitz together cottage cheese, roasted strawberries, chia seeds, a sweetener like an agave or stevia, and ice cubes. Pour the smoothie into a glass and enjoy your breakfast.

Vegetable burger and raw salad for lunch – cook a ready-to-eat vegetable or red lentil burger till brown on both sides. Chop up some favorite vegetables like cucumber, tomatoes, cabbage, and baby spinach and make a salad with a simple lime juice and agave dressing. Enjoy your lunch of vegetable burger and salad.

Roast dinner – In a greased baking pan, place potatoes, butternut pumpkin, zucchini, carrots, corn, onions, and garlic and sprinkle some rosemary. Cover the pan with aluminum foil and bake at 180C in a preheated oven for about 30 minutes. Remove the vegan roast from the packet and rub with olive oil, rosemary, and mint. Once the veggies have cooked for 30 minutes, place the roast in the middle, add some capsicum and bake for another half hour. Serve with garlic bread and mushroom gravy.

Day 16

Raspberry-banana smoothie for breakfast – In a food processor, blend together 1 large, ripe banana (frozen), 1 ¼ cup raspberry (frozen), ¾ cup orange juice, ½ cup pomegranate juice, and ¾ cup unsweetened almond milk. Your raspberry-banana smoothie is ready.

Sweet corn and cauliflower soup for lunch – In a big saucepan, put the ½ head of cauliflower (cut into florets), kernels from 2 corn cobs, 1 large potato (diced), 1 small leek, 1 tbsp. of vegetable stock, salt, and pepper and one liter of water. Bring this mixture to a boil and then simmer on a low flame for about 15-20 minutes till veggies are cooked. Cool and then blend in a food processor. Serve hot with crusty bread.

Spaghetti Bolognese for dinner – In a large saucepan, fry onions and garlic with some oil till soft. Now add mushrooms, zucchini, and carrots, stir gently and cook for 2-3 minutes. Now add canned tomatoes, anchovy-free Worcestershire sauce, tomato paste, stock cube, and herbs and mix well. Season the mixture with salt and pepper. Simmer for about 20 minutes. Cook and drain spaghetti as directed on the packet and serve with the sauce.

Chapter 5: Meal Plan and Recipes for Block III

Day 17

Peach Oat Smoothie for breakfast – In a blender, blitz together 2 ripe peaches (cut into cubes), 1 tbsp. chia seeds, ½ frozen banana, ¼ cup oats, ½ cup almond milk (unsweetened), ¼ orange juice, and agave (if you want). Your peach oat smoothie is done.

Stir Fry Veggies and Tempeh with rice for lunch – Take oil in a large pan and stir fry vegetables of your choice such as broccoli florets, carrots, zucchini, mushrooms, onions, and whatever else you like. Add spices like curry powder, cumin powder, and coriander powder and continue to stir fry like veggies are tender. Add some tempeh (cut into squares) and then add a mixture of soy sauce and sweet chili sauce. Toss everything together and serve on a plate of steamed hot rice.

Soy strips Rougaille with a watercress salad for dinner – In a large pan, heat some oil and sauté onions, garlic, thyme, and some ginger. Add tomato paste, tomatoes, and some chili and let it simmer for 2 minutes. In another pan, fry marinated soy strips in olive oil till brown. To the simmering sauce add the fried soy strips with some water and bring to a boil. Then reduce the heat and allow it to simmer for about 10 minutes or till the sauce thickens. For the watercress salad, toss together chopped watercress, carrots, and capsicum along with vinaigrette of orange juice, salt, and pepper. Place the salad on a plate and over this place the sauce-filled soy strips. Enjoy your dinner

Day 18

Banana bread smoothie for breakfast – Place 1 frozen banana, ½ cup quinoa (cooked), 1 tbsp. walnuts. 2 tbsp. flaxseed, 1 mejdul date, ¾ tsp cinnamon powder, and some ice cubes. Blitz together, pour into your glass and enjoy your smoothie.

Crispy Mock Chicken with Potato Mash for lunch – Cut "mock" chicken into chunks or strips and put them into a Ziploc pouch along with seasoning and breadcrumbs for about 30 minutes. Heat some oil in a pan, and fry this in batches till golden brown. Serve on a plate of hot mashed potatoes.

Avocado on Toast – Take a slice of your favorite bread and toast with some vegan margarine till golden brown. Pile mashed avocados over this and enjoy a healthy and extremely easy-to-make vegan lunch. You could add some sprouts and raw veggies for some crunch.

Day 19

Green Apple and Cucumber Smoothie for breakfast – In a blender, blitz together chopped green apple, 1 tbsp. walnuts, ½ a cucumber, ¼ an avocado (chopped), some agave (if you want), and ice cubes. Your delicious green apple and cucumber smoothie is ready.

Enchiladas and Guacamole for lunch – First make some chili non-carne as described in an earlier meal plan day. Get yourself some ready made tortillas and salsa. On a tortilla, spread some chili non-carne, and fold it over. Bake till the tortillas are slightly brown. Remove from the oven and place some salsa on top. Serve hot with some guacamole

Bombay potatoes with pita bread for dinner – Heat the packet of Bombay potatoes and cook as directed. Warm the pita bread and spread the potatoes and layer the top with some vegan sour cream and some fresh coriander. Dig right in.

Day 20

Strawberries smoothie for breakfast – Place 1 cup frozen strawberries, some chia seeds, some flaxseed, oats, apple cider vinegar, vanilla extract, and some ice cubes. Blitz all together and your smoothie is ready.

Roasted vegetable lasagna for lunch – In a baking dish, put together chopped eggplant, capsicum, zucchini, and onions. Drizzle some olive oil and season with salt and pepper. Toss them together and bake in a medium oven until tender. Once this is cooled, add pesto, chopped tomatoes, and tomato paste and mix thoroughly.

Make a white sauce with vegan margarine, flour, and vegan cream cheese. Now, take a baking dish, make a vegetable layer at the bottom; next place a lasagna sheet, and then pour the white sauce over. Repeat this layering process till the ingredients are all used up. Bake for about 30-40 minutes till the top is lightly brown. Enjoy your vegan lasagna hot.

Day 21

Green Smoothie for breakfast – Blend together 1 cucumber (diced), 3 cups of spinach (raw), 2 cups melon (cubed), some green tea, a little lemon juice (for tartness), some agave (if you want), and some ice cubes. Once nicely blended pour into a glass and enjoy your breakfast.

Stir-fry vegetables with marinated soy strips for lunch – In a large pan, with a little oil, stir-fry all your favorite veggies along with some marinated soy strips. Add spices and sauces of your choice. Serve on a plate of hot steamed rice.

Vegan hot dogs for dinner – Cook the readymade vegan hot dogs by boiling, steaming, or frying. Spread vegan margarine on one side of the bun (cut in half), smear mustard on the other half, place the hot dogs in the middle, and pile on cucumbers and tomato slices and some lettuce leaves. Bring the two halves of the bun together and your dinner is ready.

Day 22

Mint and chocolate chip smoothie for breakfast – Place a peppermint tea in boiling water and get a nicely concentrated cup of peppermint tea ready. In a blender, put together 1 cup unsweetened almond milk, 1 frozen banana, 2 cups of spinach, 1 tsp of hemp seeds, 2 tbsp. of chocolate chips, and ice cubes. Blitz everything and pour into a glass. Put some more chocolate chips on top and your breakfast is ready.

Thai noodles for lunch – Cook vermicelli noodles as directed on the packet. Drain and keep aside. Heat some olive oil in a large pan and add chopped veggies like celery, bok choy, spring onions, mushrooms, peanuts, chili, ginger, and garlic. Cook till the vegetables are tender. Make a mixture of light soy sauce and sesame oil. Once the vegetables are nicely tender, stir in the noodles and add the sauce mixture. Mix well. Remove from heat and serve hot.

Sandwich with soy strips for dinner – Make a yummy sandwich with your favorite bread slices and marinated soy strips. Add some raw vegetables for some crunch. You can use vegan margarine and Dijon mustard as spreads and dig right in.

Day 23

Apple Smoothie for breakfast – Blitz together 1 apple, ½ cup cherries, ½ cucumber, ½ cup raspberries, 1 tsp chia seeds, and some ice cubes. Pour into your favorite glass and enjoy the apple smoothie.

Borscht for lunch – Cook and peel beetroots. Grate half of it and thinly slice the remaining. In a large pan, heat oil, and add chopped celery, carrots, mushrooms, leeks and some water. Bring to a boil; add the grated beets, reduce the heat and simmer for about 10 minutes. In another pan, take some more water and boil the sliced beets and simmer on a medium heat for not more than 10 minutes. Drain out the beetroot slices (which you can discard) and pour the beetroot-infused juice into the other simmering veggie mixture. Remove from heat. Season with spices of your choice and your yummy borscht is ready.

Vegan prawns and some salad for dinner – In a hot skillet, fry the mock prawns with some oil. Sprinkle soy sauce. Serve hot with crunchy veggies.

Chapter 6: Meal Plan and Recipes for Block IV

Day 24

Blueberries smoothie for breakfast – This needs a little bit of planning the night before. Combine 1 ½ cups of any non-dairy milk, 2 tbsp. of oats, 1 tsp of vanilla protein powder, a little vanilla extract and 1 tsp of chia seeds. Place in the fridge the night before. In the morning, blitz this mixture along with ½ cup blueberries and your smoothie is ready.

Tempeh Cottage Pie for lunch – Fry cumin seeds, onions, garlic, and capers till tender. Put in the tempeh and fry for a couple of minutes more. Add carrots, tomatoes, corn, peas, and sweet potato and cook for another 2-3 minute. Add water and tomato paste; bring to a boil, reduce heat and simmer till the liquid reduces. But ensure that the mixture does not get too dry. Add salt and pepper for seasoning.

Nicely Mash par-boiled potatoes with soymilk and vegan margarine. Season this with salt and pepper. Pour the tempeh mixture onto a baking tray and even spread it out. Spread the mashed potato mixture over this layer and sprinkle paprika over the potatoes. Bake in a medium oven for 45 minutes till the potato layer is golden brown.

San Choy Bow for dinner – In a large wok, stir-fry onion, and garlic over a high heat. Add ginger, chili, and mushrooms and continue stir-frying for another 3 minutes. Mix in the vegan mince and stir-fry for some more minutes breaking down the lumps in the mince as you go along. Add stock and bring to a boil. Reduce heat and continue to simmer till the stock is fully absorbed. Stir in coriander, soy sauce, and some lime juice. Serve hot on a platter of lettuce leaves.

Day 25

Raspberry lemon smoothie for breakfast – This requires you to prepare the ingredients the night before. Combine 1 ½ cups of non-dairy milk, 1/ cup of raspberry, 2 tbsp. oats, 1 tbsp. lemon juice, 1 tbsp. of chia seeds, 1 tbsp. of almond butter, a little lemon zest, vanilla extract, and stevia powder. Place in the fridge overnight. In the morning, blitz this mixture in a blender till smooth. Your smoothie is ready

Vegetable curry with rice for lunch – In a pan, heat some vegetable oil, and fry onions, garlic, and cumin seeds till onions are translucent. Add chopped vegetables including potatoes, cauliflower, carrots, mushrooms, French beans, and peas. Add curry paste, turmeric powder, and coriander powder. Sprinkle a little water and cook till the veggies are tender right through. Season the curry with salt and pepper. Serve hot on a layer of steamed rice.

Potato and vegetable salad for dinner – Steam potatoes and keep aside. Make a sauce with Dijon mustard and vegan mayonnaise. Cut the potatoes and stir in some grated carrots and finely chopped onions. Stir in the sauce. Mix thoroughly and your salad is ready to be polished off.

Day 26

Blueberry peach smoothie for breakfast – Blend together 1/2 a peach, 1 cup blueberries, 1 scoop protein powder, 1 cup green tea, 1 tsp chia seeds, 1 serving probiotics, and come ice cubes in a blender till smooth. Enjoy your breakfast.

Stuffed tofu turkey for lunch – You will need a large amount of firm tofu (about 2 kg). Crumble the firm tofu and add a marinade consisting of tamari oil, olive oil, and 2 cloves of crushed garlic. Stir well and keep aside. Tightly pack this tofu in a cheesecloth-lined colander and place cheesecloth over this too. Place a heavy object on top of this arrangement and let it rest for about an hour.

For the stuffing, fry onions, garlic, mushrooms, and celery in sesame oil. Add rosemary, thyme, dried sage, black pepper, and some soy sauce and cook till the vegetables are soft. Remove from heat. Add some breadcrumbs and mix well.

Remove the heavy object and the cheesecloth from the top of the tofu arrangement. Using a big ladle, scoop out tofu from the top such that about an inch of tofu is left on three sides. Press the stuffing into this hollow and put back the scooped tofu on top and press down firmly on all sides. Turn this over onto a greased baking dish and remove the other cheesecloth too. Bake the stuffed tofu for an hour until the top is nice and brown. Remove from the oven and cool. Your stuffed tofu is ready to be carved.

Zucchini fritters for dinner – Cut zucchini into baton shapes. Make a batter with plain flour and season this with salt and pepper. Make a mixture of breadcrumbs and herbs. Dip the zucchini into the batter, then line with the breadcrumb mixture and deep fry in hot oil. Serve hot with any sauce or chutney.

Day 27

Pumpkin banana smoothie for breakfast – Blend together 1 cup almond milk, ½ banana, ½ cup canned pumpkin, ½ tsp maple syrup, vanilla extract, a little ground ginger, a pinch of all spice powder, and ice cubes in a food processor. When a smooth thick consistency is reached, you can gulp down your smoothie.

Spanakopita for lunch – Make a filling with sautéed onions, garlic, cooked and chopped spinach, mushrooms, tofu, and some roasted pine nuts. Season the filling with salt and pepper. Use this filling to make rolls using readymade filo pastry. Place the rolls on a greased baking dish and brush them with melted margarine. Bake for about 15 minutes or until golden brown. Serve warm with a vegan dip.

Vegan sushi for dinner – Cook, rinsed sushi rice till the water is all absorbed. Stir in sugar and rice vinegar with the cooked rice and mix such that there are no lumps. Keep this aside. On a nori sheet, spread this rice evenly with enough place for any filling too. Ensure you do not fill too much as then you would not be able to roll the sheets. Using a rolling mat, roll the sushi filled nori sheet and then remove the mat and cut into bite-sized pieces.

Day 28

Caramel apple green smoothie for breakfast – In a blender, put 1 frozen apple (diced), 1 cup almond milk, 2 cups spinach, 2 tbsp. peanut butter, 2 dates, ground cinnamon, and ice cubes and blitz together. Your smoothie is ready.

Asparagus and Mushroom Risotto for lunch – In a large pan, mix water, stock powder, onion powder, mushrooms, and dried herbs. Bring it to a boil and then reduce to a simmer. In another pan, melt vegan margarine with a little olive oil on a medium heat. Cook the onions till they are translucent and then add rice and stir continuously. To this rice, add wine and stir again. When the wine is completely gone, spoon in a ladle of vegetable stock. Now add the mushroom mixture. Keep adding stock as it continuously gets absorbed. Repeat this till you get the desired risotto consistency. Serve hot.

Mexican Beans and Baked Potato for dinner – Cook potatoes in a microwave for about 5 minutes. Then cook in an oven till it is crisp on the outside and soft on the inside. Heat up the readymade Mexican beans and add a little bit of margarine. Place the beans over the cooked potatoes and enjoy your meal.

Day 29

Ultra Green smoothie for breakfast – In a food processor, place 2 cups spinach, 1 cup unsweetened coconut milk, ½ a frozen banana, ½ a frozen avocado, 2 tsp of hemp seeds, and ice cubes. Blitz all the ingredients together till you get a thick smoothie. Enjoy it.

Vegan pizza for lunch – Buy a ready-made vegan pizza base and layer it with vegan cheese, thin strips of red capsicum, green capsicum, sliced mushrooms, and olives over a layer of vegan pizza sauce. Bake for about 10-15 minutes.

Lentils, Leek, and Potato Soup for dinner – Take chopped potatoes, leeks, and ½ cup of red lentils along with water and stock powder in a large pan. Bring it to a boil and then simmer on medium heat. Once cooked and cooled, blend in a food processor. Add a little hot water if you want a thinner consistency. Season the soup with salt and pepper.

Day 30

Chocolate and Raspberry smoothie for breakfast – Blend together 1 cup almond milk, 2 cups spinach, 1 cup raspberries, 2 tbsp. shredded coconut, 1 tbsp. cocoa powder, and some ice cubes in a food processor till you get a smooth consistency. Enjoy your smoothie

Fried rice for lunch – Heat oil in a large pan and sauté chopped onions. Add finely chopped veggies of your choice included cauliflower, French beans, peas, cabbage, and corn kernels. Add a sauce mixture of soy sauce and sweet chili sauce to this and cook till the veggies are tender. Add cooked rice and toss and mix thoroughly. Season the fried rice with salt and pepper if needed. Serve hot.

Antipasto Pasta Salad for dinner – Cook the pasta as per directions on the packet. Mix together thinly diced capsicum, onions, carrots, cucumber, and olives with some balsamic vinegar and antipasto salsa. Add the cooked pasta and toss all the ingredients together. Your salad is ready.

Conclusion – How to Stay Committed

If you are trying to change your lifestyle, it calls for immense commitment and hard work. It is quite easy to fall for loopholes and give up early or even halfway through because you cannot find the energy and motivation to handle the changes. This chapter is dedicated to helping you overcome these negative thoughts and help you stay committed to the vegan cause:

Set yourself easy to achieve targets initially – Setting unachievable targets can put you off as you see yourself as a failure. Take little at a time and be motivated by your small achievements. Slowly you will see setting higher targets and achieve them too.

Keep a journal and food tracker and make diligent notes – Write down everything. From what to eat, how much you have exercised, how difficult the day was in terms of keeping you on track, what were the motivation factors, what were the de-motivation factors, and more! Make note of everything no matter how trivial it may seem. When you are looking back, these notes will come in handy and will help you correct any mistakes.

Interact with people who are also facing these challenges – We are social animals and love the sense of belonging and a sense of identity. When we reach out to people who face the same situations that we face, we find that sense of belonging and the fear that we are the only ones with problems goes away. Moreover, when we interact with other people, ideas, and best practices can be exchanged which is good for all concerned.

Remember the process of change is always difficult and painful. But, if we do not take up these challenges we will stagnant which is the beginning of any end. You must steel yourself and work hard for a better tomorrow. When you are feeling low, think of the potential positive results of your endeavors and be motivated by those images and thoughts.

So, pick up the shovel, roll up your sleeves, take a firm stand, and start work immediately and be rest assured that you will find happiness, contentment and an amazing sense of achievement at the end of this seemingly arduous journey.

Help me improve this book

While I have never met you, if you made it through this book I know that you are the kind of person that is wanting to get better and is willing to take on tough feedback to get to that point. You and I are cut from the same cloth in that respect. I am always looking to get better and I wish to not just improve myself, but also this book. If you have positive feedback, please take the time to leave a review. It will help other find this book and it can help change a life in the same way that it changed yours. If you have constructive feedback, please also leave a review. It will help me better understand what you, the reader, need to make significant improvements in your life. I will take your feedback and use it to improve this book so that it can become more powerful and beneficial to all those who encounter it.

http://viewbook.at/veganbook

REMEMBER TO JOIN THE GROUP NOW!

If you have not joined the Mastermind Self Development group yet, now is your time! You will receive videos and articles from top authorities in self development as well as a special group only offers on new books and training programs. There will also be a monthly member only draw that gives you a chance to win any book from your Kindle wish list!

If you sign up through this link http://www.mastermindselfdevelopment.com/specialreport you will also get a special free report on the Wheel of Life. This report will give you a visual look at your current life and then take you through a series of exercises that will help you plan what your perfect life looks like. The workbook does not end there; we then take you through a process to help you plan how to achieve that perfect life. The process is very powerful and has the potential to change your life forever. Join the group now and start to change your life!
http://www.mastermindselfdevelopment.com/specialreport

You will also love these other great titles from Mastermind Self Development!

You will want to check out these other great titles Mastermind Self Development. All available in the Kindle store or you can just click on covers below.

http://viewbook.at/selflove

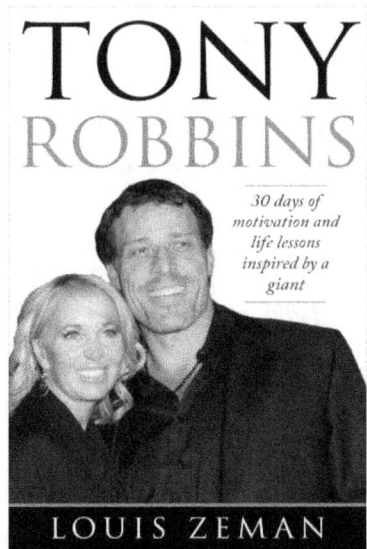

http://getbook.at/tonyrobbins

You can also find these titles by searching them in the Kindle store on Amazon.

www.ingramcontent.com/pod-product-compliance
Lightning Source LLC
Chambersburg PA
CBHW081409070526
44583CB00020B/2738